Best Diet for Life

A Weigh to Health

Special Edition

Paddleduck #4

Aunt Julie

THIS BOOK IS INFORMATION ON A JOURNEY
TO HEALTH AND WEIGHT LOSS.

**SEE YOUR DOCTOR BEFORE STARTING ANY
HEALTH OR WEIGHT LOSS PLAN.**

I have been watching my diet for years. I have tried all types of diets. They all work. Eat healthy, exercise, and watch your portions. All the diets and everything I have read took me back to the basics. I learned about proper nutrition in elementary school. My friends wanted to know how I was losing weight and liked the food I was cooking. I decided to write down and share it in a book.

Eat Healthy,

Julie Kidd Pierce

Cover Designs by Andrea Donlevy, Interior Artwork by Kandy Koehn Reddoch, Kylie Pope, and Emma Riedel.

Thank you, great job!

Best Diet for Life: A Weigh to Health - Special Edition

See other books from Aunt Julie at www.paddleduck.com.

Lulu.com Publishing

Order this book online at www.lulu.com or info@PADDLEDUCK.com

Most PADDLEDUCK titles are also available at major online book retailers.

ISBN: 978-1-105-34942-3

The Top 5 Healthiest Fat-Burning Foods

By Mike Geary, Certified Personal Trainer, Certified Nutrition Specialist, The Truth about Six Pack Abs

Grass-fed beef or bison, the typical beef or bison that you see at the grocery store is raised on grains such as corn and soybeans. Soy and corn are NOT the natural diet of cattle or bison, and therefore change the chemical balance of fats and other nutrients in the beef or bison. Grain-fed beef and bison are typically WAY too high in omega-6 fatty acids and WAY too low in omega-3 fatty acids. Grass-fed beef from cattle and buffalo (or bison) that were raised on natural foods that they were meant to eat in nature (grass and other forage), have much higher levels of healthy omega-3 fatty acids and lower levels of inflammatory omega-6 fatty acids compared to grain fed beef or bison. Grass-fed meats also typically contain up to three times the Vitamin E as grain fed meats.

Additionally, grass-fed meat from healthy cattle or bison also contain a special healthy fat called conjugated linoleic acid (CLA) in MUCH higher levels than grain-fed meat. CLA has been proven in scientific studies in recent years to help in burning fat and building lean muscle which helps you lose weight. These benefits are on top of the fact that grass-fed meats are some of the highest quality proteins that you can eat. This also aids in burning fat and building lean muscle.

The Top 5 Healthiest Fat-Burning Foods (cont'd)

Avocado, even though these are typically thought of as a "fatty food," it's all healthy fat. This fruit is also super-high in mono-unsaturated fat, but also full of vitamins, minerals, micronutrients, and antioxidants. The quality dose of healthy fats and other nutrition you get from avocados helps your body to maintain proper levels of hormones that help with fat loss and muscle building. Eating avocados helps to reduce your appetite in the hours after your meal.

Whole Eggs including the yolk (not just egg whites) Eggs are one of the highest quality sources of protein. The egg yolks are the healthiest part of the egg. That is where most of the vitamins, minerals, and antioxidants (such as lutein) are found. Egg Yolks contain more than 90% of the calcium, iron, phosphorus, zinc, thiamin, B6, folate, and B12, and panthothenic acid of the egg. The yolks contain ALL of the fat-soluble vitamins A, D, E, and K in the egg, as well as ALL of the essential fatty acids. Choose free-range organic eggs. Similar to the grass-fed beef, the nutrient content of the eggs and the balance between healthy omega-3 fatty acids and inflammatory omega-6 fatty acids (in excess) are controlled by the diet of the chickens. Chickens that are allowed to roam free outside and eat a more natural diet will give you healthier, more nutrient-rich eggs, with a healthier fat balance.

The Top 5 Healthiest Fat-Burning Foods (cont'd)

Nuts, Walnuts, Almonds, Pecans, Macadamia, etc. This "fatty food" can help you burn fat. Nuts are healthy fats, along with high levels of nutrition such as vitamins, minerals, and antioxidants.

Nuts are also a good source of fiber and protein, which helps to control blood sugar and can aid in weight loss. Nuts help to maintain good levels of fat burning hormones in your body as well as help to control appetite and cravings, so that you essentially eat less calories overall, even though you're consuming a high-fat food. Some healthy nuts are pecans, almonds, and walnuts; buy a variety, you increase the types of vitamins and minerals and the balance of polyunsaturated to monounsaturated fats you obtain. Try to find raw nuts instead of roasted nuts; it helps to maintain the quality and nutritional content of the healthy fats that you will eat.

Berries include blueberries, strawberries, raspberries, and even the "exotic" Goji berry. Berries are a powerhouse of nutrition and are packed with vitamins and minerals, and some of the best sources of antioxidants of any food in existence. Berries also pack a healthy dose of fiber, which slows your carbohydrate absorption and digestion and controls your blood sugar levels to help prevent insulin spikes (which can stimulate fat gain). Goji berries are one of the most nutrient-dense berries on the planet.

Top 15 Fat Burning Foods from eHow

When you eat these foods, your metabolism increases and helps burn away excess fat that your body is storing.

Fruits not only burn fat but also help hydrate your system:

Apples
Blackberries
Blueberries
Cherries
Cranberries
Grapes
Honeydew Melon

Vegetables

Asparagus
Broccoli
Cabbage
Carrots
Cauliflower
Cucumbers
Peppers
Pumpkin

Studies show that shellfish such as lobster and crab are also fat burning foods.

More about Fat Burning Foods

Asparagus contains the chemical asparagine.
This alkaloid stimulates the kidneys and improves the circulatory process. These alkaloids directly affect the cells and break down fat. It also contains a chemical that helps to remove waste from the body by breaking up the oxalic acid; this acid tends to glue fat to cells. By breaking the acid up, it helps reduce fat levels.

Beets are a strong diuretic that focuses on the liver and kidneys. Beets flush out floating body fats. They have a special iron that cleanses the corpuscles; corpuscles are blood cells that can contain fat deposits and also contain chlorine that will help to flush out fatty deposits. This chlorine stimulates the lymph, which will clear out the fat deposits.

Brussel sprouts stimulate the glands,
has a cleansing effect on the cells and minerals stimulate the kidneys. Waste is released quickly and helps to clean out cells.

Cabbage cleanses your body of waste matter is a
.diuretic cabbage and will help break up the fat.

Carrots contain carotene, a form of Vitamin A.
The carotene will be transformed into vitamin A in the intestines and this process will speed up your metabolism.

Fat Burning Food (cont'd)

Cucumbers' hard skin is rich in fiber and contains a variety of beneficial minerals including silica, potassium, and magnesium. These minerals work to stimulate the kidneys to wash out uric acid, which is a waste product. This in turn stimulates the removal of fat and loosens the fat from the cells.

Garlic is a natural diuretic. Garlic has mustard oils and these oils create a cleansing action in the body. This loosens fat and helps wash out the fats.

Onions, like garlic have minerals and oils that will help to breakdown fat deposits and speed up your metabolism. Eat raw onions every day; they have more power than garlic and a milder smell.

Radishes scrub the mucous membrane of your body from high levels of Iron and Magnesium. These minerals actually help to dissolve fat in the cells.

Tomatoes have high Vitamin C and Citricmalic-oxalic acids. The acid accelerates the metabolic process.

Apple Cider Vinegar

Use this diuretic in small quantities.

You can add it to your salad as a dressing.

It is made from apples and the malic acid in apples will create a fat burning process.

It is a powerful diuretic.

The fermentation process causes the vinegar to have constructive acids that join with alkaline elements and minerals in the body.

This produces a cell scrubbing effect.

It also contains high levels of potassium, which has an antiseptic quality that helps to eliminate fat deposits.

Benefits of Regular Exercise

Reduces your risk of heart disease, high blood pressure, osteoporosis, diabetes, and obesity.

Keeps joints, tendons and ligaments flexible, which make it easier to move around.

Reduces some of the effects of aging.

Contributes to your mental well-being and helps treat depression.

Helps relieve stress and anxiety.

Increases your energy and endurance.

Helps you sleep better.

Helps you maintain a normal weight by increasing your metabolism.

Low Carb Fruits

APPLES with SKIN-7g of carbs, 50-gr portion

AVOCADO- 4g of carbs, 50-gr portion

BANANA-12g of carbs, 50-gr portion

BLACKBERRIES-5g of carbs, 50-gr portion

BLUEBERRIES-7g of carbs, 50-gr portion

CANTALOUPE MELON-4g of carbs, 50-gr portion

CHERRIES (sweet)-8g of carbs, 50-gr portion

CLEMENTINE-6g of carbs, 50-gr portion

GRAPEFRUIT- (all types)-5g of carbs, 50-gr portion

GRAPES- red or green 13g of carbs, 50-gr portion (European type such as Thompson seedless)

HONEYDEW MELON-5g of carbs, 50-gr portion

KIWI FRUIT-8g of carbs, 50-gr portion

MANGO-8g of carbs, 50-gr portion

NECTARINE-6g of carbs, 50-gr portion

ORANGES- (all varieties)-5g of carbs, 50-gr portion

PAPAYA-5g of carbs, 50-gr portion

PEACH-5g of carbs, 50-gr portion

PEAR-7g of carbs, 50-gr portion

PERSIMMON-9g of carbs, 50-gr portion

PINEAPPLE-6g of carbs, 50-gr portion

PLUMS-6g of carbs, 50-gr portion

RASPBERRIES-6g of carbs, 50-gr portion

STRAWBERRY-4g of carbs, 50-gr portion

TANGERINE-8g of carbs, 50-gr portion

WATERMELON-4g of carbs, 50-gr portion

Low Carb Vegetables

ARUGULA-1g of carbs, 50-gr portion

ASPARAGUS (boil, drain, no salt)-2g of carbs, 50-gram portion

BEETS (canned)-4g of carbs, 50-gr portion

BROCCOLI (boil, drain, no salt)-4g of carbs, 50-gr portion

CABBAGE-3g of carbs, 50-gr portion

CARROT-5g of carbs, 50-gr portion

CAULIFLOWER-3g of carbs, 50-gr portion

CELERY-2g of carbs, 50-gr portion

CUCUMBER (peeled)-1g of carbs, 50-gr portion

GREEN, SNAP/STRING BEANS-4g of carbs, 50-gr portion

GREEN, SWEET/BELL PEPPER-2g of carbs, 50-gr portion

KALE-5g of carbs, 50-gr portion

LETTUCE (iceberg)-2g of carbs, 50-gr portion

LETTUCE (romaine)-2g of carbs, 50-gr portion

OKRA (boil, drain, no salt)-2g of carbs, 50-gr portion

ONIONS (all types)-7g of carbs, 50-gr portion

RADISHES-2g of carbs, 50-gr portion

RED, SWEET or BELL PEPPER-3g of carbs, 50-gr portion

SNOW or SUGAR SNAP PEAS-5g of carbs, 50-gr portion

SPINACH-4g of carbs, 50-gr portion

SWEET CORN-10g of carbs, 50-gr portion

TURNIPS (boil, drain, no salt)-2g of carbs, 50-gr portion

WHITE MUSHROOMS-2g of carbs, 50-gr portion

Dr. Perricone's Super foods

There are more than 10 "super foods." In fact, just about every brightly colored fruit and vegetable fits the category of a super food, as do nuts, beans, seeds and aromatic and brightly colored herbs and spices. The beneficial properties of each one of these super foods could fill an entire book.

The 10 featured here were chosen because of their direct link to the Brain-Beauty Connection. These foods (listed here in alphabetical order) are rich in the Essential Fatty Acids (EFAs), antioxidants or fiber, and as in the case of açaí—all three.

In addition, we have included foods that have been proven to lower or help regulate blood sugar levels, an extremely important factor for all of those concerned with slowing the aging process and preventing diabetes, obesity, wrinkles, and a host of degenerative diseases.

Acai Berry is a super food.

Anything in the "Alliums Family" Garlic, onions, leeks, scallions, chives, and shallots can all help the liver eliminate toxins and carcinogens.

Barley can be used as a breakfast cereal, in soups and stews, and as a rice substitute. Barley is also high in fiber, helping metabolize fats, cholesterol, and carbohydrates.

Dr. Perricone's 10 Super foods (cont'd)

Green Foods, wheat and barley grasses can be bought in powder, tablet, or juice form and offer greater levels of nutrients than green leafy vegetables. They also help cholesterol, blood pressure, and immune response.

Buckwheat: Seed and Grain, buckwheat is loaded with protein, high in amino acid, stabilizes blood sugar, and reduces hypertension.

Beans and Lentils, you can reduce cholesterol while beefing up on antioxidants, folic acid, and potassium. Try kidney, black, navy, pinto, chickpeas, soybeans, peas, and lentils.

Hot Peppers, both bell and chili peppers contain antioxidants, have twice the Vitamin C as citrus fruit, and work as great fat burners.

Nuts and Seeds, you cannot go wrong with a handful of nuts a day—walnuts, hazelnuts, almonds, macadamia, and pistachio nuts contain omega-3.

Sprouts, numerous varieties of sprouts are great with any meal. Great source of protein.

Yogurt and Kefir, these cultured foods contain healthful bacteria that aid immune function and the calcium helps burn fat. Try using them as a base for a smoothie.

Fats and Oils, Omega-3 fatty acids are found in cold-water oily fish, flax seeds, and canola oil and pumpkin seeds. Consumption of monounsaturated fats found in olive oil, avocado, and nuts has been linked to reduced risk of cardiovascular disease. Other healthful oils include rice bran oil, grape seed oil, and walnut oil.

Fruits and Vegetables
Whole fruits, berries and vegetables are rich in vitamins, minerals,
fiber, antioxidants, and phytochemicals. Choose green and brightly colored vegetables, and whole fruits. You should eat at least five (and preferably more) servings of fruits and vegetables each day.

Protein Sources. Possible anti-inflammatory protein sources include lean poultry, fish, and seafood (fatty fish offer protein as well as omega-3 fatty acids). Soy and soy foods such as tofu and tempeh, along with other legumes, can be used as plant-based protein sources.

Beverages. Your body needs water. Drink tap, sparkling or bottled water, 100% fruit juice, herbal tea, low-sodium vegetable juice and low-or non-fat milk.

Anti-inflammatory Diet Tips

When you are choosing anti-inflammatory foods, choose fresh foods instead of heavily processed foods.

Here are some tips:

For breakfast, try oatmeal served with fresh berries and walnuts.

Snack on whole fruits, nuts, seeds, and fresh vegetables instead of cookies and candy.

Eat more fish and less fatty red meat.

Cook with olive oil and canola oil.

Try a tofu stir-fry or scramble.

Have a salad with lots of fresh vegetables as your meal.

Stay away from deep-fried foods; bake, broil, poach or stir-fry instead.

Choose dark green or brightly colored vegetables as side dishes --they should fill half your dinner plate.

Drink water, non-fat milk, 100% fruit and vegetable juices, herbal and green tea instead of sugary sodas and soft drinks.

Pro-Inflammatory Foods to Avoid

- Breads, rolls, baked goods, bagels, croissants, crackers, corn bread, corn muffins, muffins

- Candy, cake, cookies

- Cereals (except old-fashioned oatmeal)

- Cornstarch

- Corn syrup

- Doughnuts

- Egg rolls

- Fast food, french fries

- Fruit juice

- Fried foods

- Flour

- Granola

- Hard cheese (except for feta and grating cheeses)

- Honey

- Hot dogs

- Ice cream, frozen yogurt, italian ices

- Jams, jellies and preserves

- Margarine

Pro-Inflammatory Foods to Avoid (cont'd)

- Molasses

- Noodles

- Pancakes, pastry, pie, pita bread, pizza, pasta

- Popcorn

- Potatoes

- Pudding

- Relish

- Rice

- Sherbet

- Shortening

- Snack foods, including potato chips, pretzels, corn chips, rice and corn cakes, etc.

- Soda

- Sugar

- Tacos

- Tortillas

- Waffles

6 Essential Flat-Belly Foods

Eat This, Not That by David Zinczenko, with Matt Goulding a Yahoo-Health Expert for Nutrition

Quinoa Per ¼ cup: 170 calories 2.5 g fat 7 g protein 3 g fiber. For starters, anytime you choose a whole-grain product over one made from nutrient-stripped white flour, you wage war against belly fat. Penn State researchers found that dieters who ate whole-grains lost twice as much belly fat as those who stuck to white-flour products—even though they had consumed the same number of calories. What's more, quinoa contains twice the belly-filling protein as regular cereal grains, fewer glucose-raising carbohydrates, and even a handful of healthy fats. So start your day off with a cup of cooked quinoa combined with a ½-cup of milk and ½ cup of blueberries—microwave for 60 seconds, and you have a delicious (and slimming) alternative to your traditional oatmeal.

Green Tea 0 calories. Catechins, the powerful antioxidants found in green tea, are known to increase metabolism. A study by Japanese researchers found that participants who consumed 690 milligrams of catechins from green tea daily had significantly lower body mass indexes and smaller waist measurements than those in a control group. It is safe to say that green tea is one of the best beverages for your health.

6 Essential Flat-Belly Foods (cont'd)

Kefir   Per cup: 174 calories 2 g fat 14 g protein 3 g fiber. Think of kefir as drinkable yogurt, or an extra-thick, protein-packed smoothie. This delicious dairy product is a belly-blasting essential. Beyond the satiety-inducing protein, the probiotics in kefir may also speed weight loss. British scientists found that these active organisms boosted the breakdown of fat molecules in mice, preventing the rodents from gaining weight.

Avocado   Per avocado: 322 calories 29 g fat (4 g saturated, 20 g monounsaturated) 13 g fiber 4 g protein. Never fear this full-fat Mediterranean-diet staple: It is teeming with healthy monounsaturated fats (also found in olive oil), which have been linked to lowered LDL cholesterol levels and weight loss. A study in The New England Journal of Medicine found that the healthy-fat Mediterranean diet was more effective than a diet that avoided fats.

Eggs   Per one large egg: 102 calories 7 g fat (2 g saturated) 7 g protein. A British study found that people who increased the percentage of protein-based calories in their diet burned 71 more calories a day

Grapefruit   Per grapefruit: 104 calories 4 g fiber   2 g protein. A grapefruit a day in addition to your regular meals can speed weight loss. The fruit's acidity slows digestion, it takes longer to move through your system, you will end up feeling fuller, and more satisfied, for longer. Vitamin C-packed grapefruit works to lower cholesterol and decrease risk of stroke, heart disease, and some types of cancer.

Anti-Aging Foods

All these anti-aging foods contain antioxidants or other substances that help your body repair damage and stay young.

Green tea is an ancient drink for health and longevity.

Antioxidants in **dark chocolate** protect your heart against aging, damage, and heart disease.

Apples reduce the risk of metabolic syndrome.

Lycopene is a substance in **tomatoes** for anti-aging.

Fish are a great source of protein and healthy fats.

Red wine's properties can extend longevity and life span.

Beans provide a big supply of antioxidants that prevent damage by free radicals.

Water can be healthy and even "detox" your body.

Vegetables are a source of nutrients and antioxidants. They help you lose weight and help your body repair and live longer.

Melons are a delicious source of vitamins and other nutrients.

Walnuts are a great anti-aging food because of the amount of omega-3s in just a handful. They prevent dementia and keep your brain young while fighting off heart disease by improving your cholesterol.

More Information on ANTI-AGING FOODS

The general guidelines for the anti-aging diet: keep your calorie consumption and saturated fat intake down, eat plenty of wholegrain, oily fish and fresh fruit and vegetables, and cut down on salt and sugar. In addition to these general guidelines, there are specific foods that have a role in anti-aging and that you should regularly include in your diet.

Avocado, this fruit, which is usually eaten as a vegetable, is a good source of healthy monounsaturated fat that may help to reduce levels of a bad type of cholesterol in body. Avocado is a good source of vitamin E and can help to maintain healthy skin and prevent skin aging (vitamin E may also help alleviate menopausal hot flashes). It is rich in potassium, which helps prevent fluid retention and high blood pressure.

Berries, all black and blue such as blackberries, blueberries, black currants and black grapes contain phytochemicals known as flavonoids-powerful antioxidants which help to protect the body against damage caused by free radicals and aging.

Cruciferous vegetables include cabbage, cauliflower, broccoli, kale, turnip, brussel sprouts, radish, and watercress. These assist the body in its fight against toxins and cancer. If possible, eat them raw or very lightly cooked so that the important enzymes remain intact.

More on ANTI-AGING FOODS (cont'd)

Garlic, eating a clove of garlic a day helps to protect the body against cancer and heart disease. The cardio protective effects of garlic are well recorded. One 1994 study in Iowa, USA, of 41,837 women between the age of 55 and 69 suggested that women who ate a clove of garlic at least once a week were 50 percent less likely to develop colon cancer. Another study at Tasgore Medical College in India suggested that garlic reduced cholesterol levels and assisted blood thinning more effectively than aspirin, thus helping to reduce the risk of heart disease.

Ginger, this spicy root can boost the digestive and circulatory systems, which can be useful for older people. Ginger may also help to alleviate rheumatic aches and pains.

Nuts, most varieties of nuts are good sources of minerals, particularly walnuts and brazil nuts. Walnuts, although high in calories, are rich in potassium, magnesium, iron, zinc, copper, and selenium. Adding nuts to your diet can enhance the functioning of your digestive and immune systems, improve your skin, help to control, and prevent cancer. Nuts may also help control cholesterol levels.

Soya, menopausal women might find that soya helps to maintain estrogen levels. Soya may alleviate menopausal hot flash and protect against Alzheimer's disease, osteoporosis and heart disease.

More on ANTI-AGING FOODS (cont'd)

Look out for fermented soya products. They are more easily digested, more nutritional, and do not generally cause food intolerances. You may want to check that soya products have not been genetically modified. Soya should not be confused with soya sauce, which is full of salt and should be used sparingly, if at all.

Whole meal pasta and rice, complex carbohydrates provide a consistent supply of energy throughout the day and should make up the bulk of your diet. Whole meal pasta is an excellent complex carbohydrate. It is high in fiber and contains twice the amount of iron as normal pasta. Brown rice is another recommended complex carbohydrate, which is high in fiber and B vitamins.

http://www.womenfitness.net

NEGATIVE CALORIE FOODS

* Apples

* Asparagus

* Beets

* Berries (blue, cranberries, raspberries, strawberries)

* Broccoli

* Cantaloupes

* Carrot

* Cauliflower

* Celery stalk, celery root

* Cucumbers

* Eggplant

* Endives

* Garlic

* Grapefruit

* Green beans

* Green cabbage

* Lamb's lettuce, lettuce

* Lemons

NEGATIVE CALORIE FOODS (cont'd)

* Onions

* Papayas

* Pineapples

* Prunes

* Radishes

* Spinach

* Tangerines

* Tomatoes

* Turnips

* Zucchini

LONGEVITY FOODS

These food and drink options will help your body fight off the damage caused by aging. They will help your body fight age-related illnesses.

Avocados are loaded with healthy fats to help improve your cholesterol

Walnuts are a great (and mercury-free) source of omega-3 essential fatty acids

Green Vegetables can decrease heart disease, cancer, high blood pressure and more. Focus on leafy or deeply colored vegetables for the most benefit.

Water has no calories.

Berries are packed full of antioxidants and other chemicals that your body can use to make repairs and prevent some of the damage caused by aging.

Green Tea has been a longevity supplement in Asia for thousands of years. Green tea contains high concentrations of just the chemicals your body needs. Green tea gives a mild (and gentle) energy boost from its caffeine.

Red Wine is good for you and contains a substance called "resveratrol" that helps your body fight off age-related illnesses.

Beans are a great source of healthy protein and antioxidants.

LONGEVITY FOODS (cont'd)

Melons have some of the best nutritional profiles of all the fruits. They are pulpy (so they fill you up) and contain many vitamins for your body.

Dark Chocolate is last in this list only because it does not need to be higher up to get your attention. Chocolate (dark chocolate that is) is good for you. It has a balance of fats that do not harm your body and tons of healthy chemicals that your body needs. The only drawback is that chocolate also has calories. Have a little square every day, but do not overdo it.

http://longevity.about.com/od/lifelongnutrition/tp/top-anti-aging-foods.htm

Boost Immunity & Stay Healthy -Antioxidants and Your Immune System

One of the best ways to keep your immune system strong and prevent colds and flu might surprise you: Shop your supermarket's produce aisle. Experts say a diet rich in fruits and vegetables can help you ward off infections like colds and flu. That is because these super foods contain immune-boosting antioxidants. What are antioxidants? They are vitamins, minerals, and other nutrients that protect and repair cells from damage caused by free radicals. Many experts believe this damage plays a part in a number of chronic diseases, including hardening of the arteries (atherosclerosis), cancer, and arthritis. Free radicals can also interfere with your immune system. So fighting off damage with antioxidants helps keep your immune system strong, making you better able to ward off colds, flu, and other infections. Adding more fruit and vegetables of any kind to your diet will improve your health. The three major antioxidant vitamins are beta-carotene, vitamin C, and vitamin E. You will find these in colorful fruits and vegetables – especially those with purple, blue, red, orange, and yellow hues. Beta-carotene and other carotenoids: Apricots, asparagus, beets, broccoli, cantaloupe, carrots, corn, green peppers, kale, mangoes, turnip and collard greens, nectarines, peaches, pink grapefruit, pumpkin, squash, spinach, sweet potato, tangerines, tomatoes, and watermelon.

Boost Immunity & Stay Healthy -Antioxidants and Your Immune System (cont'd)

Vitamin C: Berries, broccoli, brussel sprouts, cantaloupe, cauliflower, grapefruit, honeydew, kale, kiwi, mangos, nectarines, orange, papaya, red, green or yellow peppers, snow peas, sweet potato, strawberries, and tomatoes.

Vitamin E: Broccoli, carrots, chard, mustard and turnip greens, mangoes, nuts, papaya, pumpkin, red peppers, spinach, and sunflower seeds.

Other super foods that are rich in antioxidants include:

- Prunes

- Apples

- Raisins

- All berries

- Plums

- Red grapes

- Alfalfa sprouts

- Onions

- Eggplant

- Beans

Boost Your Brain

Almonds and blueberries lower blood sugar. Healthy snacks can improve cognition. In this case, the omega-3s in the almonds and the antioxidants in the blueberries can keep your brain functioning correctly.

Walnuts, Omega-3's in walnuts have been found to improve mood and calm inflammation. They also replace lost melatonin, which is necessary for healthy brain functioning.

Sodium-free alternative for salt, hypertension can lead to heart problems, but new evidence suggests that decreasing the salt in your diet can also improve blood flow to the brain and decrease dementia.

Drink two cups of **gotu kola tea** daily, this ayurvedic herb, used for centuries in India, regulates dopamine. Dopamine in the brain helps protect brain cells from harmful free radicals, boosts pleasurable feelings, and improves focus and memory.

Try some new tea, **Tulsi tea**, made of an Indian herb called holy basil, and ginseng tea, both contain herbs that can help reduce overproduction of the stress hormone cortisol, which can hamper memory. The herbs also help keep you alert.

Sip red wine, up to two glasses for women and up to three for men weekly delivers the powerful antioxidant resveratrol, which may prevent free radicals from damaging brain cells. Beware: Drinking more than that could leach thiamine, a brain-boosting nutrient.

Boost Your Brain (cont'd)

Pears, apples, oranges, and cantaloupe, the combination prevents elevated blood sugar that could impede brain cells from firing correctly. It also provides fiber and antioxidants that help scrub plaque from brain arteries and mop up free radicals that inhibit clear thinking.

Rolled oats with cinnamon, the oats scrub plaques from your brain arteries, while a chemical in cinnamon is good for keeping your blood sugar in check—which can improve neurotransmission.

Curry, the active ingredient in Indian curry, turmeric, contains resveratrol, the same powerful antioxidant that makes red wine good for brain health. Curry protects brain cells from harmful free radicals.

Salmon and sardines, check that the fish is from the wild, not domestically raised. They keep your heart-and brain-healthy.

Sleep is when your brain consolidates memories. Poor sleep, caused by medical conditions, worry, depression, or insomnia, can interfere with your rest. So treat yourself to relaxing scents like vanilla before bed. They raise the chemical dopamine and reduce cortisol, a stress hormone.

20 Super Foods for Weight Loss

Eat More To Weigh Less, by Dean Ornish.

Steak has a reputation as a diet buster, but eating it may help you peel off pounds. In a study published in The American Journal of Clinical Nutrition, women on a diet that included red meat lost more weight than those eating equal calories but little beef. "The protein in steak helps you retain muscle mass during weight loss," says study author Manny Noakes, Ph.D. Try to consume local organic beef; it is healthier for you and the environment. Grill or broil 4-ounces.

Egg, yolks and all, they will not harm your heart, and they can help you trim inches. Women on a low-calorie diet who ate an egg with toast and jelly each morning lost twice as many pounds as those who had a bagel for breakfast with the same number of calories but no eggs, reported a study from LSU in Baton Rouge. "Egg protein is filling, so you eat less during the day.

Kale, one raw chopped cup contains 34 calories and about 1.3 grams of fiber, as well as a hearty helping of iron and calcium. Spinach is another nutrient powerhouse.

Oats "Oatmeal has the highest satiety ranking of any food," Grotto says. "Unlike many other carbohydrates, oats—even the instant kind—digest slowly, so they have little impact on your blood sugar." All oats are healthful, but the steel-cut and rolled varieties have up to 5 grams of fiber per serving, the most filling choice.

Lentils are a true belly flattener. "They're high in protein and soluble fiber, two nutrients that stabilize blood sugar levels," says Tanya Zuckerbrot, R.D., author of The F-Factor Diet. "Helps prevent insulin spikes that cause your body to create excess fat in the abdominal area."

Goji berries have a hunger-curbing edge over other fruit: 18 amino acids, which make them a surprising source of protein, say Chef Sarah Krieger, R.D., spokesperson in St. Petersburg, Florida, for the ADA.

Wild salmon, heart healthy and they shrink your waist. "Omega-3 fatty acids improve insulin sensitivity which helps build muscle and decrease belly fat," Grotto explains. The more muscle you have, the more calories your body burns. Wild salmon may contain fewer pollutants.

Apple a day can keep weight gain at bay, finds a study from Penn State at University Park. People who chomped an apple before a pasta meal ate fewer calories overall than those who had a different snack. "Apples are high in fiber—4 to 5 grams each—which makes them filling," says Susan Kraus, R.D., a clinical dietitian at Hackensack University Medical Center in New Jersey. The antioxidants in apples may help prevent metabolic syndrome, a condition marked by excess belly fat or an "apple shape."

Buckwheat pasta is high in fiber and contains protein. Zuckerbrot says, "Those two nutrients make it very satiating, so it's harder to overeat buckwheat pasta than the regular pasta."

Blueberries have the highest antioxidant level of all commonly consumed fruit, according to research from the USDA Agriculture Research Service in Little Rock, Arkansas. They also deliver 3.6 grams of fiber per cup. "Fiber may actually prevent some of the fat you eat from being absorbed because fiber pulls fat through the digestive tract," Zuckerbrot says.

Almond butter may lower bread's glycemic index (a measure of a food's effect on blood sugar). A study from the University of Toronto found that people who ate almonds with white bread did not experience the same blood sugar surges as those who ate only the slice. "The higher blood sugar levels rise, the lower they fall; that dip leads to hunger, causing people to overeat," says study author Cyril Kendall, Ph.D. "Furthermore, blood sugar changes cause the body to make insulin, which can increase abdominal fat."

Pomegranate juice gets all the hype for being healthy, but pomegranate seeds deserve their own spotlight. In addition to being loaded with folate and disease-fighting antioxidants, they are low in calories and high in fiber, so they satisfy your sweet tooth without blowing your diet, Krieger says. Eat the raw seeds or toss in a salad.

Chile Pepper cranks up your metabolism. "A compound in the pepper called "capsaicin" has a thermogenic effect, meaning it causes the body to burn extra calories for 20 minutes after you eat peppers," Zuckerbrot explains. Plus, "you can't gulp down spicy food," she adds. "Eating slowly gives your brain time to register that your stomach is full, so you won't overeat."

Yogurt has carbs, protein and fat, and can stave off hunger by keeping blood sugar levels steady. In a study from the University of Tennessee at Knoxville, people on a low-calorie diet that included yogurt lost 61 percent more fat overall and 81 percent more belly fat than those on a similar plan but without yogurt.

Quinoa can curb hunger and is as easy as piling your plate with this whole grain. It packs fiber (2.6 grams per 1/2 cup) and protein, a great nutrient combo that can keep you satisfied for hours.

Sardines are high in protein and loaded with omega-3's, which also help the body maintain muscle. They are low in mercury and high in calcium.

Tarragon can use this herb in place of salt in marinades and salad dressings. Excess sodium causes your body to retain water, so using less salt can keep bloating at bay.

Parmesan, women who had one serving of whole milk or cheese daily were less likely to gain weight over time, a study in The American Journal of Clinical Nutrition finds. Whole dairy may have more conjugated linoleic acid, which might help your body burn fat.

Avocado makes a top weight loss food, Kraus says. The heart-healthy monounsaturated fat increases satiety.

Olive oil has healthy fat that increases satiety, taming your appetite. Research shows it has anti-inflammatory properties. Chronic inflammation in the body is linked to metabolic syndrome.

Super Health with Super Foods

Hass Avocados are rich in the good fat, commonly known as monounsaturated and higher in potassium than a banana. High in Vitamins E and B6, fiber and folate, they contain both cholesterol lowering and cancer protecting nutrients.

Blueberries are a small blue fruit that packs a mighty punch to your health. High in antioxidant power, thanks to the anthocyanins that give them their beautiful color, blueberries are also high in ellagic acid (a cancer preventive) and tannins (fights urinary tract infections). One cup of blueberries can provide you with nearly 4 grams of fiber and a healthy dose of Vitamin C.

Broccoli is a super food. High in sulforaphane and indole-3-carbinol, this great green veggie could help to modify natural estrogens and increase enzyme activities that could destroy cancer-causing cells. Eating three servings of broccoli or any of its friends (bok choy, brussel sprouts, cauliflower, or cabbage) will help to keep you healthy.

Butternut Squash is not a vegetable but a fruit. A great source of beta-carotene, just one cup of cooked squash can give you more than four times the daily-recommended dose of Vitamin A. Surprisingly high in calcium, that same one cup can give you 10 percent of the daily-recommended amount of this bone-building mineral.

Flaxseed is a seed from the flax plant. High in protein, fiber, and Omega 3 fatty acids.

Super Health with Super Foods (cont'd)

Flaxseed is also a great source for lignans, which are proving to help prevent hormone-related cancers. They can be ground into flour, easily added to anything you bake.

Kale is the unsung hero of the green leafy vegetables. For years, treated as nothing more than garnish, kale is now coming into its own. High in antioxidants including lutein and zeacanthin, it is fast becoming a tasty way to help protect your vision.

Kiwi fruit, technically a berry, has proven to be one of the most nutritious foods available. Just two medium kiwis have more potassium than a banana and twice as much vitamin C and fiber as an orange. All that is in addition to the Vitamin E, copper, lutein, folate, and magnesium that also is power packed into this small fruit.

Lentils All vegetarians know that adding lentils to their menu helps to replace the meat protein missing from their diets. What they may not realize is that lentils also offer an incredible amount of healthy nutrients. Jam-packed with heart protecting folate, fiber, protein, and iron, they cook up in a snap with no pre-soaking needed and come in a wide variety of colors.

Yogurt is known for its healthy properties. It provides a wonderful source of protein and calcium, as well as the friendly bacteria that aids in good digestion and helps to boost immunity.

10 Everyday Super Foods

Yogurt, low fat or fat-free plain yogurt is higher in calcium than some other dairy products and contains protein and potassium. "Yogurt can be enriched with probiotics for a healthy balance of bacteria in your gut, and beneficial, heart-healthy plant stanols," says Zied. "And lactose sensitive people may tolerate yogurt better than milk." Look for plain yogurt fortified with vitamin D, and add your own fruit to control sweetness and calories. Skim milk is another super dairy food that has only 83 calories per cup and is easy to slip into coffee to help you get one of the recommended three servings of dairy each day. "Dairy foods contain practically every nutrient you need for total nutrition --and in just the right balance," says bone health expert, Robert Heaney, MD.

Eggs make the list because they are nutritious, versatile, economical, and a great way to fill up on quality protein. "Studies show if you eat eggs at breakfast, you may eat fewer calories during the day and lose weight without significantly affecting cholesterol levels," says Elizabeth Ward, MS, RD, author of The Pocket Idiot's Guide to the New Food Pyramids. Eggs also contain 12 vitamins and minerals, including choline, which is good for brain development and memory.

Nuts have a high fat content but their protein, heart-healthy fats, high fiber, and antioxidant content are healthy. Today Show nutritionist Joy Bauer, MS, RD says that nuts in small doses help lower cholesterol levels and promote weight loss.

10 Everyday Super Foods (cont'd)

Kiwi is among the most nutritionally dense fruit, full of antioxidants, says Ward. "One large kiwi supplies your daily requirement for vitamin C," says Ward. "It is also a good source of potassium, fiber, and a decent source of vitamin A and vitamin E, which is one of the missing nutrients. Kiwifruit can also have a mild laxative effect due to their high fiber content.

Quinoa is one of the best whole grains you can eat, according to Zied. "It is an ancient grain, easy to make, high in protein (8 grams in 1 cup cooked), fiber (5 grams per cup), and a naturally good source of iron," she says. "Quinoa (pronounced keen-wa) also has plenty of zinc, vitamin E, and selenium to help control your weight and lower your risk for heart disease and diabetes," she says. Quinoa is as easy to prepare as rice and can be eaten alone or mixed with vegetables, nuts, or lean protein for a whole-grain medley. Try to make at least half your daily grain servings whole grains.

Beans are loaded with insoluble fiber, which helps lower cholesterol, as well as soluble fiber, which fills you up and helps rid your body of waste. They are also a good, low-fat source of protein, carbohydrates, magnesium, and potassium. Joy Bauer favors edamame (whole soybeans) because they also contain heart-healthy omega-3 fatty acids.

10 Everyday Super Foods (cont'd)

Salmon is a super food because of its omega-3 fatty acid content. Studies show that omega-3 fatty acids help protect heart health. That is why the American Heart Association recommends eating fatty fish like salmon twice weekly. Salmon is low in calories (200 for 3 ounces) and lots of protein, is a good source of iron, and is very low in saturated fat. (Mercury is known to accumulate in fish.)

Broccoli is one of America's favorite vegetables because it tastes good and is available all year long. It is a rich source of vitamin A, vitamin C, and bone-building vitamin K, and has plenty of fiber to fill you up and help control your weight.

Sweet potatoes are a delicious member of the dark orange vegetable family, which lead the pack in vitamin A content. Substitute a baked sweet potato (also loaded with vitamin C, calcium, and potassium) for a baked white potato. Before you add butter or sugar, taste the sweetness when a sweet potato is cooked. You save calories over that loaded baked potato.

Berries pack an incredible amount of nutritional goodness into a small package. They are loaded with antioxidants, phytonutrients, low in calories, and high in water and fiber to help control blood sugar, and keep you full longer. Their flavors satisfy sweet cravings. Blueberries lead the pack because they are among the best source of antioxidants and are widely available.

Top 10 Ways to Boost Your Energy

WebMD Weight Loss Clinic-Feature

Increase Your Magnesium Intake

Walk around the Block

Take a Power Nap

Don't Skip Breakfast --or Any Other Meal

Reduce Stress and Deal with Anger

Drink More Water and Less Alcohol

Eat More Whole Grains and Less Sugar

Have a Power Snack

Make It a Latte

Check Your Thyroid Function and

Complete Blood Cell Count

Benefits of Water,

An increased intake of healthy water will greatly enhance digestion, nutrient absorption, skin hydration, detoxification and virtually every aspect of better health. So many common ailments and illnesses can be prevented with an increased intake of healthy water. Headaches, hypertension, back pain, arthritis, ulcers, asthma, morning sickness, and fatigue can all benefit and in many cases be prevented by regulating the body's natural fluid levels. With the proper intake of healthy water and the right minerals and nutrients, our body can overcome almost anything. An increased intake of water and the proper immune enhancing nutrients combined with a little patience and common sense are the best defense against most infections. Fluids and rest increase our natural resistance.

The best offense is a good "defense." Our brain is over 75% water and when it detects a shortage of available fluids, it implements a water rationing process by producing histamines, causing pain and fatigue. This natural process is meant to slow us down and conserve water. Histamines are released as a warning signal that something is wrong. When we take antihistamines or analgesic medicines like acetaminophen or ibuprofen, we simply turn off the signal and often allow the problem to progress.

Natural Diuretics

Apple cider vinegar maintains the potassium levels.

Artichokes

Asparagus contains asparagine -a chemical alkaloid that boosts kidney performance, thereby improving waste removal from the body.

Beets attack floating body fats and fatty deposits.

Brussel Sprouts help in stimulating the kidneys and pancreas.

Cabbage is known to breakdown fatty deposits especially around the abdominal region.

Carrots are a rich source of carotene that speed the metabolic rate of the body and hasten removal of fat deposits and waste.

Cranberry juice can aid removal of excess fluid retention.

Cucumbers are rich in sulfur and silicon that stimulate the kidneys into better removal of uric acid and help increase urination and better flushing out of toxins.

Dandelion leaf tea aids in detoxification.

Garlic aids breakage of fat.

Green tea has been in use for centuries in China.

Horseradish, radish, and raw onions will speed up metabolism.

Lettuce aids metabolism and eliminates toxins.

Tomatoes are rich in Vitamin C that aid the metabolism and release of water from the kidney to flush out waste.

Watercress

Watermelons increase urination and eliminate toxins.

Calorie and Nutritional Comparison of Snacks

Snack (typical serving size)	Calories	Fat (g)	Carbs (g)	Protein (g)
Cucumber Slices (1/2 cup)	6.8	0.1	1.4	0.4
Carrot Sticks (1/2 cup)	27.5	0.1	6.5	0.7
Tangerine Slices (1 large)	43.1	0.2	11	0.6
Applesauce (1/2 cup)	52.5	0.1	13.8	0.2
Celery w/Cr Che (1 Tbsp)	54.4	5.1	1.3	1.3
Grapes (1/2 cup)	56.8	0.5	14.2	0.5
Dried Apricots (1/4 cup)	77.4	0.1	20.1	1.2
Apple Slices (1 med)	81.4	0.5	21	0.3
Pretzels (1 oz.)	108	1	22.5	2.6
Oil-Popped Popcorn (2 cups)	110	6.2	12.6	2
Graham Crackers (2 large)	118.5	2.9	21	1.9
Jelly Beans (30)	121.1	0.2	30.7	0
Raisins (1/4 cup)	123.8	0.2	32.6	1.3
Trail Mix (1 oz.)	131	8.3	12.7	3.9
BBQ Chips (1 oz.)	139.2	9.2	15	2.2
Tortilla Chips (1 oz.)	142	7.4	17.8	2
Cheese n Crackers (1 oz.)	142.6	7.2	16.5	2.9
Chocolate Pudding (1/2 cup)	150.3	4.5	25.8	3.1
Cheese Puffs (1 oz.)	157.1	9.8	15.3	2.2
Cashews (1 oz.)	162.7	13.1	9.3	4.3
Sunflower Seeds (1 oz.)	165	14.1	6.8	5.5
Peanuts (1 oz.)	165.8	14.1	6.1	6.7
Colby Cheese Cubes (1.5 oz.)	167.5	13.7	1.1	10.1
Beef Jerky (1.5 oz.)	174.4	10.9	4.7	14.1
Apple Slices w/PB(1 Tbsp)	176.3	8.7	24.1	4.3
Chocolate Bar (1.55 oz.)	225.7	13.5	26	3
Choc. Chip Cookies (4 med)	236.2	10.8	32.7	2.4
Doughnut (1)	250.2	11.9	34.4	2.7
Chocolate Ice Cream (1 cup)	285.1	14.5	37.2	5
Fig Bars (6)	334.1	7	68.1	3.6
French Fries (med order)	458.3	24.7	53.3	5.8

Foods that make you feel full

These foods can help curb hunger and cut your calorie intake By Theresa Stahl, RD, LDN

Beans (soy, lentils, kidney, black, garbanzo, pinto, etc.)

Protein foods such as fish, poultry without skin and lean meats

Low fat or skim milk or soymilk or low fat, low-sugar yogurt

Eggs or egg whites

Oatmeal

Whole grain cereals and breads

Fruits

Vegetables

Salads (go easy on dressings)

Soups (broth-based)

How to Rev Up Your Metabolism from eHow.com

One of the keys to weight loss and more energy is to rev up your metabolism.

Things you will need:

Protein-rich foods that is low in fat

Clean drinking water

Green juice or green juice powder

Oatmeal

Protein-rich snacks such as nuts

Start out by eating a protein-rich breakfast very shortly after waking. This jump-starts your body for the day.

Oatmeal is a great addition to your protein choice as it helps to cleanse your body and reduce cholesterol.

Make sure you include some aerobic activity as early in the morning as possible. This also wakes up your body and increases your metabolic rate.

Drink 6 to 8 glasses of water a day to help carry toxins away that can make you sluggish.

Eat a protein-rich snack at least every three hours; this will keep your body from entering a "starvation" mode, which slows down metabolic rate.

Include weight-bearing exercise at least twice a week. Muscle burns fat and increases metabolism.

Boost your fat burning process

Reduce your calorie intake by 10%-15%. The formula is simple, you eat less = you weigh less. A dramatic reduction of your calorie intake can lower your metabolism, causing your body to survive with fewer calories than before. If you moderately reduce the calorie intake, your body will have less food to "burn" and it will be forced to use your body fat and you will then have enough energy to exercise.

Replace some complex carbohydrates with vegetables.

Instead of eating one cup of rice, eat 2 cups of broccoli or 1-cup broccoli with 1/2 cup rice. Vegetables are usually low in calories.

Eat good fats - Most dieters avoid fats because 1 g of fat has more calories than 1 g of carbohydrate. Fats are good for you! Omega-3 fatty acids cannot be synthesized by the human body; this essential nutrient must be obtained from food. You should try to limit animal fat if you have cholesterol problems and introduce virgin oil (olives or grapes), nuts, or fish into your meals. The second problem is that people tend to over-eat carbs like rice, pasta, grains, and potatoes.

Get with your doctor and figure out how many calories you need to eat daily for better health and split your meals into 5 - 6 smaller meals.

Boost your fat burning process (cont'd)

Do not skip meals; you may eat more when you do eat.

Reduce animal fats. In order to lose body fat you have to reduce your calorie intake and one way you can do that is choosing leaner meat and low fat dairy products.

Increase the protein intake. The RDA's (Recommended Daily Allowance) recommendation for protein is 0.8 g/kg. If you exercise heavily you might need to increase your protein intake to 1.5-2 g/kg. This is because resistance training and endurance workouts can rapidly break down muscle protein.

Drink water because a dehydrated body can cause a slow metabolism. Drink enough water to be hydrated, but do not overdo it.

Coffee is not for everybody, so you should check with your doctor before using coffee. It takes less than an hour on average for caffeine to begin affecting the body and a mild dose wears off in three to four hours.

Do not eat too much before bedtime. Big meals before bedtime will transform into fat because your body cannot consume all the calories you have eaten. Try to eat a small protein meal instead.

Spice it up. Red Chile pepper and other hot spices can increase your metabolism. Adding hot peppers to your food can increase the body's fat burning process.

Weight Loss Tips

When you think you are hungry, drink a big glass of water. Sometimes we are really just thirsty.

"Studies show people who eat 4-5 meals or snacks per day are better able to control their appetite and weight," says obesity researcher Rebecca Reeves, Dr PH, RD.

Protein is the ultimate fill-me-up food; it is more satisfying than carbs or fats and keeps you feeling full longer. It also helps preserve muscle mass and encourages fat burning.

"Add spicy peppers to your food for a flavor boost. If you eat food that is loaded with flavor you will stimulate your taste buds and be more satisfied, you won't eat as much," says American Dietetic Association spokesperson Malena Perdomo, RD.

Having ready-to-eat snacks and meals-in-minutes on hand sets you up for success. Here are some essentials to keep on hand: frozen vegetables, whole-grain pasta, reduced-fat cheese, canned tomatoes, canned beans, pre-cooked grilled chicken breast, whole grain tortillas or pita bread, and bags of salad greens

Eat less pasta or bread and more veggies. "You can save from 100-200 calories if you reduce the portion of starch on your plate and increase the amount of vegetables," says Cynthia Sass, RD, a spokesperson for the American Dietetic Association.

TEN WARDROBE STAPLES FOR WOMEN

Whether you are at your ideal weight or not, you want to look good! Use these classic staples to build or boost your wardrobe.

Classic pencil or A-line skirt: the pencil skirt creates curves on a thin woman and accentuates curves on a curvier woman. The trick to a great pencil skirt is the fit and length. It should fit snugly but comfortably through the hip and thigh, and hit just at the knee. If you are not comfortable in a figure-hugging pencil skirt, try an A-line skirt that hits at or just above the knee.

Well-fitting jacket: A well-fitting jacket can be paired with a skirt or pants for work, or used to dress up a pair of jeans. When choosing a jacket make sure it buttons comfortably at your natural waist.

A pair of flats and a pair of heels: Basic black is always safe, especially if you have a conservative work environment.

Jeans: A dark wash in a fit that flatters your figure is the best way to go when choosing jeans. Look for jeans that fit well through the hip and then have the waist and leg length tailored. A tip on jeans from *What Not to Wear*, if you find jeans in a fit that you love, buy several pair and have the length tailored to go with different shoes of varying heights.

The little dress: Common fashion advices dictates black, but brown, dark gray or navy are also easy neutrals to accessorize. Try the shirtdress and/or the wrap dress. They flatter most figures and travel well.

White button-down shirt: The details make the difference when you are picking out a white dress shirt. You can go for a classic, tailored oxford or you can find a more feminine design that incorporates pleats, ruffles, or well-placed darts to make it more form fitting. Find a short-sleeved or sleeveless version for summer and a long-sleeved or 3/4-sleeve for winter.

Black or navy dress pants: A pair of well-tailored, trouser-cut pants in a dark color is a dressier alternative to jeans, and is great for work. A gray pinstripe is also a nice choice--neutral, but the pinstripe keeps it interesting.

Dresses: Summer in Texas means day or sundresses. In the thick heat and humidity of July, even shorts seem like too much fabric. It is getting hotter everywhere!

Cardigan sweaters: A cardigan is particularly useful here in Houston, when we move back and forth between intense heat and humidity, and frigid air conditioning all day long.

A day bag and an evening clutch: You need one of each to take you from day to night. I favor big day bags so I can fit my wallet, planner, and camera, but for my evening bag, I need only enough room for a lipstick, credit card, and some cash.

Optional accessories: Sunglasses; bangles; string of pearls; a watch; galoshes; a variety of belts (colors and sizes) a short trench coat; diamond (faux or real) studs.

WARDROBE BASICS CHECKLIST

Little Black Dress (LBD)

Black Blazer

Crisp white button down shirt

White silk t-shirt (or dressy looking t-shirt)

Black pants

Tan/khaki pants

Black knee length skirt

Tan/khaki jacket

Classic neutral color trench coat

Black leather bag

Dark denim jeans

Black pumps

1 White and 1 Black Cardigan Sweater

Pearls

Blue jean jacket

Do not wear hose with open toed shoes.

Wrap dress

REFERENCES

AMERICAN DIETETIC ASSOCIATION

DIET.COM

DR. OZ

DR. PERRICONE

FIRST FOR WOMEN

GOOD MORNING AMERICA

HEALTH

HOLISTIC HEALTH (Benefits of Water)

MAYO CLINIC

MSNBC.COM

MYDAILYMOMENT.COM

MYPYRAMID.GOV

NUTRITION.GOV

OPRAH.COM

QUALITYHEALTH.COM

REAL SIMPLE

SHAPE

SPARKPEOPLE.COM

TODAY SHOW

WOMENS FITNESS

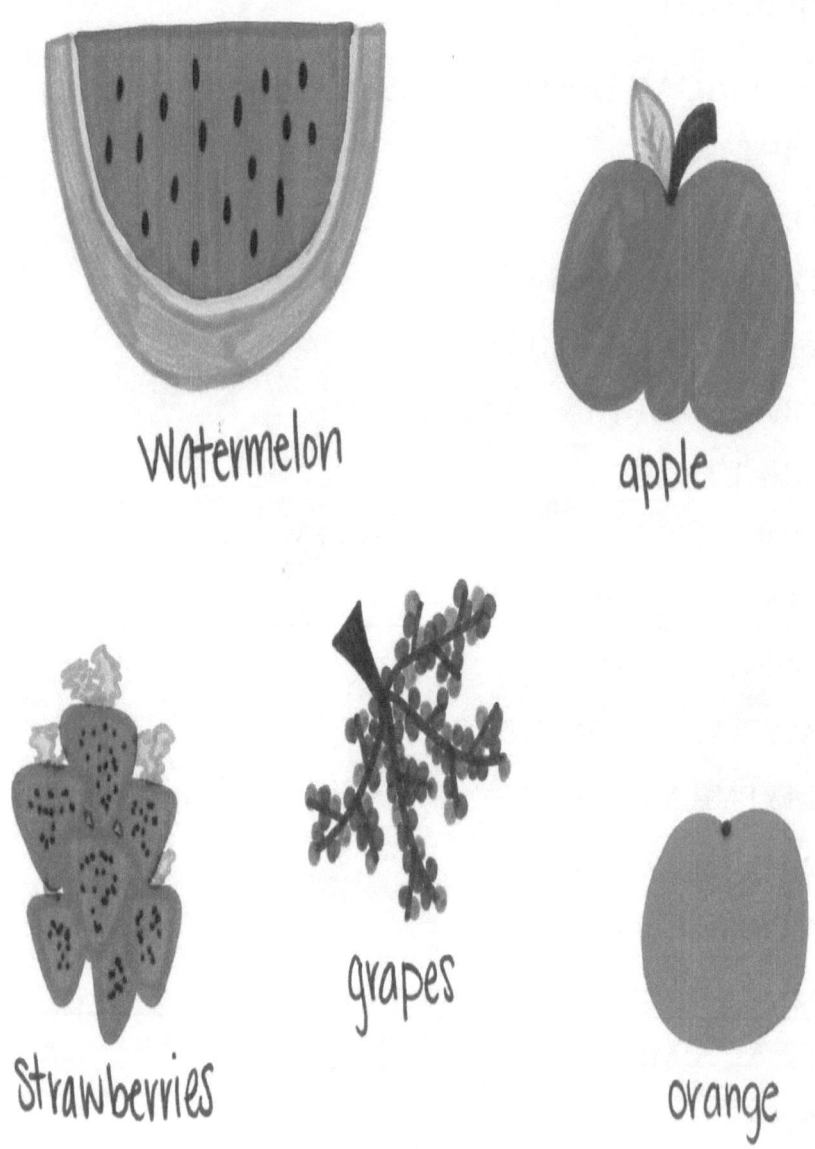

Watermelon

apple

Strawberries

grapes

orange

By Kandy Koehn Reddoch

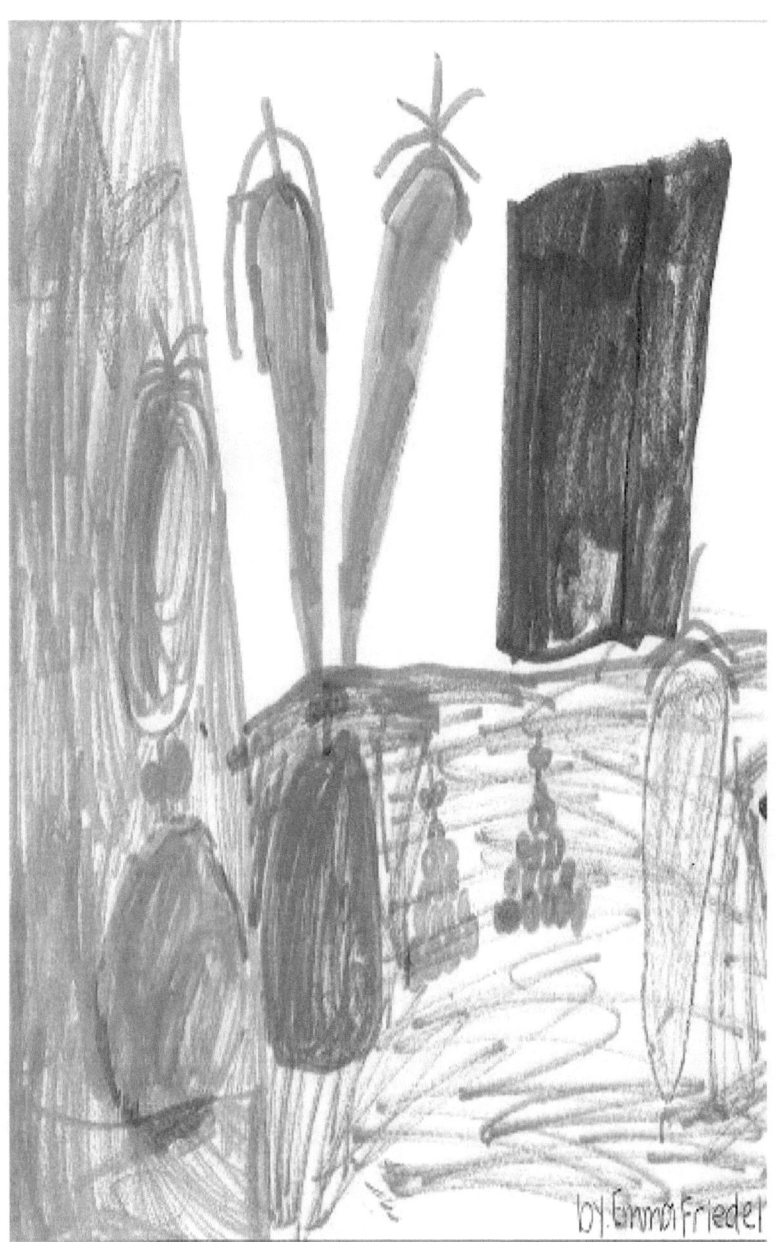

by Emma Friedel

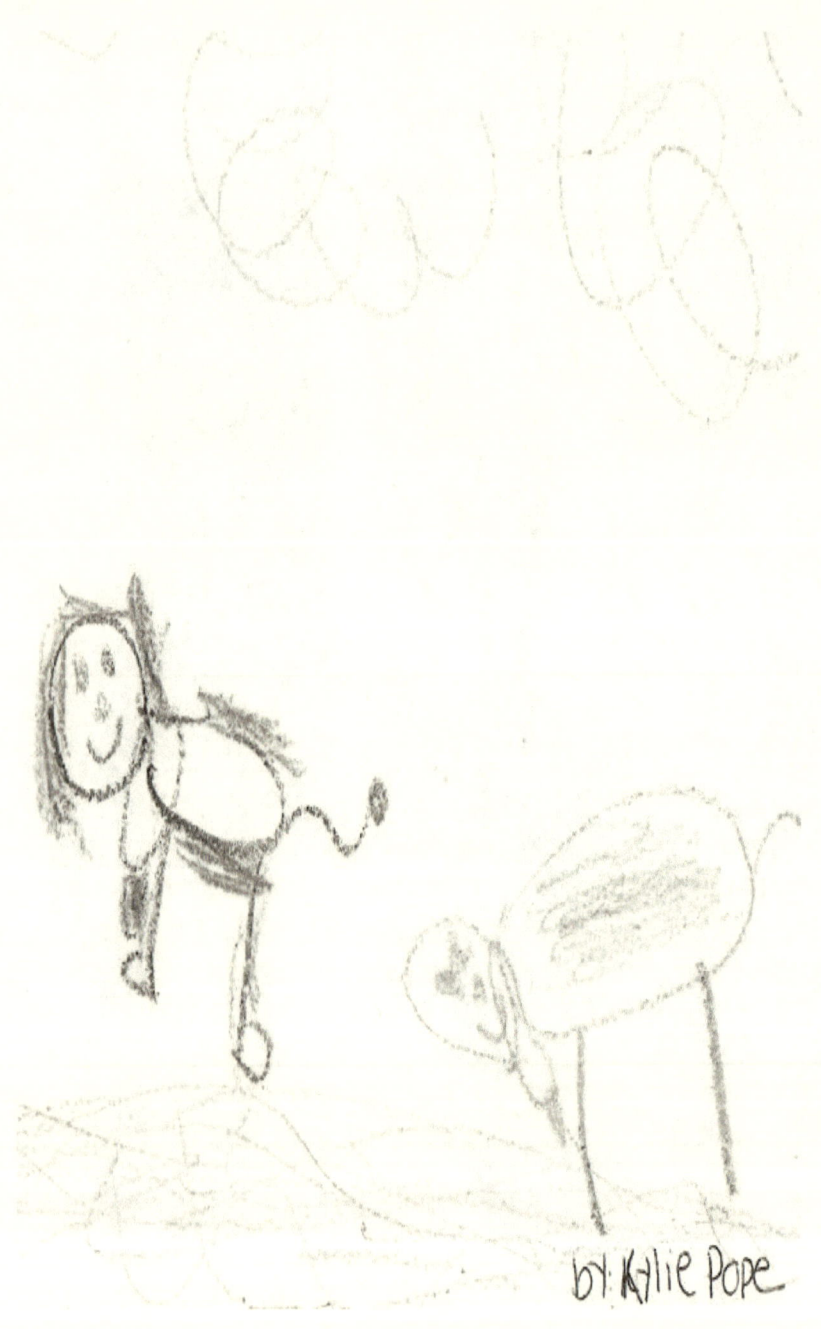

by Kylie Pope